HOW TO LOSE WEIGHT WITHOUT EXERCISE FOR MEN

Cookbook to Learn About Foods that Burn Fat.

Michael Samuel

TABLE OF CONTENTS

<u>SUCCESS STORIES AND TESTIMONIALS</u>
<u>CONCLUSION</u>

INTRODUCTION

Overview of Weight Loss Without Exercise

In the pursuit of a healthier lifestyle, many people focus on exercise as the primary method for weight loss. While physical activity is undeniably beneficial, it's not the only path to achieving and maintaining a healthy weight. For various reasons—whether due to physical limitations, busy schedules, or personal preference—some individuals may find it challenging to incorporate regular exercise into their daily routines. This book is designed for men who are looking to lose weight without the necessity of exercise, by focusing on dietary changes and nutrition.

Understanding that weight management is a multifaceted process, this guide provides comprehensive insights into how specific foods can aid in fat burning and overall weight loss. Through practical advice and delicious recipes, we aim to empower you to make healthier food choices that support your weight loss goals.

The Role of Diet in Weight Management

Diet plays a crucial role in weight management. While exercise can help burn calories, the foundation of weight loss is a caloric deficit—consuming fewer calories than your body needs to maintain its current weight. The quality of the calories consumed is just as important as the quantity. A balanced diet rich in whole, nutrient-dense foods not only supports overall health but also boosts metabolism and enhances the body's ability to burn fat.

This book will guide you through the process of choosing the right foods, understanding portion sizes, and planning meals that support weight loss. By focusing on nutrient-rich foods, you can satisfy your hunger, reduce cravings, and maintain energy levels throughout the day, all while shedding excess weight.

Understanding Metabolism and Fat Burning

Metabolism refers to the chemical processes that occur within your body to maintain life, including converting food into energy. It is often misunderstood as a simple "fast" or "slow" rate of burning calories, but in reality, metabolism encompasses a range of biochemical processes.

A key component of metabolism is the Basal Metabolic Rate (BMR), which is the number of calories your body needs to perform basic functions like breathing and digestion while at rest. Factors such as age, gender, body composition, and genetics influence BMR. While you can't change some of these factors, you can influence your metabolism through diet.

Certain foods and nutrients can enhance metabolic rate and increase fat burning. For instance, proteins require more energy to digest than carbohydrates or fats, a phenomenon known as the thermic effect of food. Additionally, some foods contain compounds that can stimulate metabolic activity and promote fat loss.

In this book, you'll learn about the foods that can help boost your metabolism and support fat burning, as well as how to incorporate them into your diet effectively. By understanding the science behind metabolism and nutrition, you can make informed choices that align with your weight loss goals, even without a traditional exercise regimen.

CHAPTER 1:

THE SCIENCE OF WEIGHT LOSS

How the Body Burns Fat

The process of burning fat, also known as lipolysis, is a critical component of weight loss. It involves the breakdown of stored triglycerides (a type of fat) in fat cells into free fatty acids and glycerol, which can then be used for energy. This process is primarily triggered when the body experiences a calorie deficit—when you consume fewer calories than your body needs for daily activities and bodily functions.

Several hormones, including insulin, glucagon, adrenaline, and norepinephrine, play key roles in regulating fat metabolism. Insulin, which is released in response to eating carbohydrates, promotes the storage of fat, whereas hormones like glucagon and adrenaline help mobilize fat stores for energy. By controlling the intake of certain nutrients and managing insulin levels, you can influence the body's ability to burn fat more efficiently.

Fat burning occurs predominantly in the mitochondria, the powerhouse of the cell, where fatty acids undergo a process called beta-oxidation. This process generates ATP (adenosine triphosphate), the primary energy currency of cells. Understanding these biochemical pathways can help you make dietary choices that favor fat oxidation, such as consuming healthy fats and proteins while moderating carbohydrate intake.

The Importance of a Balanced Diet

A balanced diet is crucial for overall health and effective weight management. It provides the essential nutrients needed for energy production, muscle maintenance, and bodily functions. A well-balanced diet typically includes a variety of macronutrients—proteins, carbohydrates, and fats—in appropriate proportions, along with vitamins, minerals, and other micronutrients.

Proteins are vital for building and repairing tissues, including muscles, which can increase your metabolic rate. They also have a high thermic effect, meaning the body uses more energy to digest them compared to fats and carbohydrates.

Carbohydrates are the body's preferred energy source, especially for the brain and muscles. However, not all carbohydrates are created equal. Whole grains, vegetables, and fruits provide complex carbs that are digested slowly, helping to maintain steady blood sugar levels and prolong satiety. In contrast, refined carbohydrates and sugars can lead to rapid spikes in blood sugar and insulin, potentially promoting fat storage.

Fats are essential for hormone production, brain function, and the absorption of fat-soluble vitamins. Healthy fats, such as those found in avocados, nuts, seeds, and olive oil, support heart health and can enhance satiety, preventing overeating.

A balanced diet also means paying attention to portion sizes and meal timing, both of which can affect metabolic rate and fat loss. This chapter will delve deeper into how to structure your diet to optimize fat burning and overall health.

Common Myths About Weight Loss

There are numerous myths and misconceptions about weight loss, often perpetuated by popular media and fad diets. Here are a few common myths debunked:

1. Myth: Skipping Meals Helps You Lose Weight Faster
   - Reality: Skipping meals can lead to overeating later and may slow down your metabolism as the body goes into conservation

mode. It's more effective to eat regular, balanced meals to keep your metabolism steady.

2. Myth: All Calories Are Equal
   - Reality: While the concept of "calories in vs. calories out" is fundamental, the source of those calories matters. For example, 100 calories from vegetables provide different nutrients and have different effects on satiety and metabolism compared to 100 calories from candy.

3. Myth: Carbs Are the Enemy
   - Reality: Not all carbohydrates are bad. Complex carbohydrates, such as those found in whole grains and vegetables, provide essential nutrients and energy. It's important to focus on the quality and quantity of carbohydrates in your diet.

4. Myth: You Can Target Fat Loss in Specific Areas
   - Reality: Spot reduction, or losing fat from specific body parts through targeted exercises, is

a myth. Fat loss occurs throughout the body as you create a calorie deficit.

5. Myth: Eating Fat Makes You Fat
   - Reality: Healthy fats are an important part of a balanced diet and can help you feel full and satisfied. The type of fat and the overall caloric balance are more important than simply avoiding fat.

Understanding these myths and focusing on scientifically backed principles can help you navigate the often confusing landscape of weight loss information. This chapter aims to provide you with the knowledge to make informed decisions about your diet and lifestyle, leading to sustainable weight loss and improved health.

CHAPTER 2:

FOODS THAT BURN FAT

Understanding Thermogenic Foods

Thermogenic foods are those that increase the body's metabolic rate, leading to an increase in calorie burning. This process is known as thermogenesis, where the body generates heat and, as a result, burns calories. The thermic effect of food (TEF) refers to the increase in metabolic rate after ingestion, digestion, absorption, and processing of nutrients. Foods with a high thermic effect require more energy to process, thereby boosting metabolism and aiding in fat loss.

Thermogenic foods often contain specific compounds that stimulate the body's metabolism. For example, capsaicin, found in chili peppers, can increase metabolic rate temporarily. Similarly, caffeine, present in coffee and tea, can enhance fat oxidation and energy expenditure. By understanding and incorporating thermogenic foods into your diet, you can naturally enhance your body's fat-burning capabilities.

Top Fat-Burning Foods and Their Benefits

Lean Proteins

Lean proteins are essential for weight loss and muscle maintenance. They have a high thermic effect, meaning the body expends more energy to digest them compared to fats and carbohydrates. Additionally, proteins are crucial for preserving muscle mass during weight loss, which helps maintain a higher metabolic rate.

Examples of Lean Proteins:
- Chicken breast
- Turkey
- Lean cuts of beef and pork
- Fish (such as salmon, tuna, and cod)
- Eggs

- Plant-based proteins (tofu, tempeh, legumes)

Benefits:
- Supports muscle maintenance and growth
- Enhances satiety, reducing overall calorie intake
- Promotes fat loss by increasing metabolism

Whole Grains

Whole grains are an excellent source of complex carbohydrates, fiber, and essential nutrients. Unlike refined grains, whole grains are digested slowly, providing a steady release of energy and preventing rapid spikes in blood sugar levels. This helps regulate appetite and reduce cravings.

Examples of Whole Grains:
- Oats
- Brown rice
- Quinoa
- Barley
- Whole wheat products (bread, pasta)

Benefits:
- Provides sustained energy and improves satiety
- Rich in fiber, aiding digestion and promoting a healthy gut
- Can help regulate blood sugar levels

Fruits and Vegetables

Fruits and vegetables are nutrient-dense and low in calories, making them ideal for weight loss. They are high in fiber, which helps you feel full longer, and are packed with vitamins, minerals, and antioxidants that support overall health. Certain fruits and vegetables also contain compounds that may enhance fat metabolism.

Examples:
- Leafy greens (spinach, kale, lettuce)
- Cruciferous vegetables (broccoli, cauliflower, Brussels sprouts)
- Berries (blueberries, strawberries, raspberries)
- Citrus fruits (oranges, grapefruits, lemons)
- Apples and pears

Benefits:
- Low in calories and high in nutrients
- Supports digestion and detoxification
- May have thermogenic properties, especially spicy vegetables like chili peppers

Healthy Fats

Healthy fats are essential for hormone production, brain function, and overall health. While fats are more calorie-dense than proteins and carbohydrates, they are crucial for a balanced diet and can aid in weight loss by promoting satiety and reducing overall calorie intake.

Examples of Healthy Fats:
- Avocado
- Nuts and seeds (almonds, chia seeds, flaxseeds)
- Olive oil
- Coconut oil
- Fatty fish (salmon, mackerel)

Benefits:

- Supports heart health and reduces inflammation
- Provides essential fatty acids for brain and cellular function
- Can improve satiety and help control appetite

How to Incorporate Fat-Burning Foods into Your Diet

Incorporating fat-burning foods into your diet can be simple and enjoyable. Here are some practical tips:

1. Plan Balanced Meals: Aim to include a source of lean protein, healthy fat, and complex carbohydrates in each meal. For example, grilled chicken (protein) with quinoa (whole grain) and a side salad with olive oil dressing (healthy fat).

2. Snack Smart: Choose nutrient-dense snacks like a handful of nuts, a piece of fruit, or vegetables with hummus. These options provide energy and essential nutrients without excessive calories.

3. Experiment with Spices: Use thermogenic spices like chili peppers, cayenne, and ginger in your cooking to boost metabolism and add flavor without extra calories.

4. Stay Hydrated: Drinking plenty of water supports metabolism and can help you differentiate between hunger and thirst. Herbal teas and green tea, which contain metabolism-boosting compounds, are also good options.

5. Prioritize Whole Foods: Focus on whole, minimally processed foods that are rich in nutrients and low in added sugars and unhealthy fats. This not only aids in weight loss but also supports overall health.

By making these foods a regular part of your diet, you can enhance your body's natural fat-burning processes and support your weight loss goals in a sustainable and healthy way.

CHAPTER 3:

MEAL PLANNING AND PREPARATION

The Importance of Meal Planning

Meal planning is a crucial component of successful weight management and healthy eating. It involves organizing your meals and snacks ahead of time, ensuring that you have nutritious options readily available. By planning your meals, you can:

1. Control Portion Sizes: Planning allows you to manage portion sizes and prevent overeating. This is particularly important for weight loss, as controlling calorie intake is key to creating a calorie deficit.

2. Make Healthier Choices: When you plan your meals, you're more likely to choose balanced,

nutrient-dense foods rather than resorting to unhealthy convenience options. It also helps you avoid last-minute decisions that might lead to less nutritious choices.

3. Save Time and Reduce Stress: By planning and preparing meals in advance, you save time during the week and reduce the stress of figuring out what to eat each day. This is especially helpful for those with busy schedules.

4. Save Money: Meal planning can help you stick to a grocery list, avoid impulse purchases, and reduce food waste. By knowing exactly what you need, you can make more efficient use of your resources.

5. Support Dietary Goals: Whether your goal is to lose weight, maintain a healthy weight, or simply eat better, meal planning helps ensure you're getting the right nutrients in the right amounts. It allows you to track your intake and adjust as needed.

Tips for Effective Meal Prep

Effective meal prep involves preparing meals and ingredients in advance, making it easier to stick to your meal plan. Here are some tips to get started:

1. Set Aside Time for Planning and Prep: Dedicate a specific day or time each week for planning your meals and doing the necessary prep work. For many, Sunday is a popular day for meal planning and prepping.

2. Create a Menu: Plan out your meals for the week, including breakfast, lunch, dinner, and snacks. Consider your schedule and plan for busy days when you might need quicker, more convenient options.

3. Make a Grocery List: Based on your menu, create a detailed grocery list. Stick to the list to avoid unnecessary purchases and ensure you have all the ingredients you need.

4. Prep Ingredients in Advance: Prepare ingredients ahead of time, such as chopping vegetables, cooking grains, or portioning out snacks. Store these prepped items in the refrigerator or freezer to keep them fresh.

5. Cook in Batches: Cook larger portions of meals and store them in individual containers for easy reheating. This is particularly useful for dinners and lunches, as it saves time and ensures you have a healthy meal ready to go.

6. Use Versatile Ingredients: Choose ingredients that can be used in multiple dishes throughout the week. For example, grilled chicken can be used in salads, wraps, or paired with different sides.

7. Invest in Quality Containers: Use good-quality, leak-proof containers to store your meals. This helps keep your food fresh and makes it easy to grab meals on the go.

8. Label and Date Your Meals: Label your containers with the name of the dish and the date it was prepared. This helps you keep track of freshness and ensures you use items in a timely manner.

Sample Meal Plans for Weight Loss

Here are two sample meal plans to give you an idea of how to structure your meals for weight loss. These plans focus on balanced nutrition, portion control, and incorporating fat-burning foods.

Sample Meal Plan 1:

Breakfast:
- Greek yogurt with mixed berries and a drizzle of honey
- A handful of almonds

Lunch:

- Grilled chicken salad with mixed greens, cherry tomatoes, cucumber, and olive oil vinaigrette
- A slice of whole-grain bread

Snack:
- Apple slices with peanut butter

Dinner:
- Baked salmon with quinoa and steamed broccoli
- A side of mixed green salad

Snack:
- A small piece of dark chocolate or a few berries

Sample Meal Plan 2:

Breakfast:
- Overnight oats with chia seeds, banana slices, and a sprinkle of cinnamon
- Green tea

Lunch:
- Turkey and avocado wrap with whole-grain tortilla, spinach, tomato, and a side of carrot sticks

Snack:
- A smoothie made with spinach, pineapple, protein powder, and almond milk

Dinner:
- Stir-fried tofu with mixed vegetables (bell peppers, broccoli, carrots) in a garlic soy sauce
- Brown rice

Snack:
- A handful of mixed nuts

These meal plans are examples of how to include a variety of nutrient-dense foods that support weight loss. Remember to adjust portion sizes and ingredients based on your specific dietary needs and preferences. By planning and prepping your meals, you can ensure that you stay on track with your weight loss goals while enjoying delicious and satisfying food.

CHAPTER 4:

BREAKFAST RECIPES

Quick and Nutritious Breakfast Options

Starting your day with a nutritious breakfast can set the tone for healthy eating throughout the day. Here are some quick and easy breakfast ideas that are both delicious and nourishing:

1. Overnight Oats
   - Ingredients: Rolled oats, Greek yogurt, chia seeds, almond milk, mixed berries, honey.
   - Instructions: In a mason jar or container, combine oats, Greek yogurt, chia seeds, and almond milk. Stir well and let it sit overnight in the refrigerator. In the morning, top with mixed berries and a drizzle of honey.

2. Avocado Toast

- Ingredients: Whole-grain bread, ripe avocado, lemon juice, salt, pepper, cherry tomatoes (optional), arugula (optional).
- Instructions: Toast the bread. Mash the avocado and mix in lemon juice, salt, and pepper. Spread the mixture on the toast. Top with sliced cherry tomatoes and arugula if desired.

3. Greek Yogurt Parfait
- Ingredients: Greek yogurt, granola, mixed fruits (such as berries, banana slices, and kiwi), honey.
- Instructions: In a bowl or glass, layer Greek yogurt, granola, and mixed fruits. Drizzle with honey. Repeat the layers if desired.

4. Egg Muffins
- Ingredients: Eggs, spinach, cherry tomatoes, bell peppers, feta cheese, salt, pepper.
- Instructions: Preheat the oven to 350°F (175°C). Whisk the eggs in a bowl and add chopped spinach, cherry tomatoes, bell peppers, and feta cheese. Season with salt and pepper.

Pour the mixture into a greased muffin tin and bake for 20-25 minutes, or until the eggs are set.

5. Banana Peanut Butter Wrap
   - Ingredients: Whole-grain tortilla, banana, natural peanut butter, chia seeds, honey.
   - Instructions: Spread peanut butter on the tortilla. Place the banana on one end and sprinkle it with chia seeds and a drizzle of honey. Roll up the tortilla and slice it in half.

High-Protein Breakfast Recipes

A high-protein breakfast helps keep you full longer and supports muscle maintenance. Here are some protein-packed breakfast ideas:

1. Scrambled Eggs with Smoked Salmon
   - Ingredients: Eggs, smoked salmon, spinach, cherry tomatoes, chives, salt, pepper.
   - Instructions: In a pan, sauté spinach and cherry tomatoes until wilted. Add beaten eggs and scramble. Top with smoked salmon and chopped chives. Season with salt and pepper.

2. Protein Pancakes

   - Ingredients: Protein powder, oats, egg whites, banana, almond milk, baking powder, vanilla extract.

   - Instructions: Blend all ingredients until smooth. Pour the batter onto a hot, non-stick skillet. Cook until bubbles form on the surface, then flip and cook until golden brown. Serve with fresh berries and a drizzle of honey.

3. Cottage Cheese and Fruit Bowl

   - Ingredients: Cottage cheese, mixed fruits (such as berries, pineapple, and mango), nuts, honey.

   - Instructions: In a bowl, add a generous serving of cottage cheese. Top with mixed fruits and nuts. Drizzle with honey.

4. Tofu Scramble

   - Ingredients: Firm tofu, turmeric, nutritional yeast, spinach, bell peppers, onion, salt, pepper.

   - Instructions: Crumble tofu in a pan and sauté with turmeric and nutritional yeast. Add chopped spinach, bell peppers, and onion. Cook until vegetables are tender. Season with salt and pepper.

5. Chia Seed Pudding with Protein Powder
   - Ingredients: Chia seeds, almond milk, protein powder, vanilla extract, fresh berries.
   - Instructions: Mix chia seeds, almond milk, protein powder, and vanilla extract in a bowl. Stir well and refrigerate overnight. In the morning, stir again and top with fresh berries.

Smoothies and Shakes

Smoothies and shakes are convenient and versatile options for a quick, nutritious breakfast. Here are some recipes to try:

1. Green Protein Smoothie
   - Ingredients: Spinach, banana, protein powder, almond milk, chia seeds, ice.
   - Instructions: Blend all ingredients until smooth. Add more almond milk if needed to reach the desired consistency.

2. Berry Blast Smoothie
   - Ingredients: Mixed berries (blueberries, strawberries, raspberries), Greek yogurt, almond milk, honey, flaxseeds.
   - Instructions: Blend the berries, Greek yogurt, almond milk, and honey until smooth. Add flaxseeds and blend briefly.

3. Chocolate Peanut Butter Protein Shake
   - Ingredients: Chocolate protein powder, banana, natural peanut butter, almond milk, ice.
   - Instructions: Blend all ingredients until smooth. For a thicker shake, add more ice.

4. Tropical Mango Smoothie
   - Ingredients: Mango, pineapple, coconut water, Greek yogurt, chia seeds.
   - Instructions: Blend the mango, pineapple, coconut water, and Greek yogurt until smooth. Stir in chia seeds and serve.

5. Oatmeal Breakfast Shake

- Ingredients: Rolled oats, banana, protein powder, almond milk, cinnamon, honey.
- Instructions: Blend rolled oats until fine. Add banana, protein powder, almond milk, cinnamon, and honey. Blend until smooth.

These breakfast recipes are designed to be nutritious, satisfying, and easy to prepare. They provide a good balance of protein, healthy fats, and complex carbohydrates, helping to fuel your day and support your weight loss goals.

CHAPTER 5:

LUNCH RECIPES

Light and Filling Lunch Ideas

A satisfying lunch is essential for maintaining energy levels and preventing overeating later in the day. Here are some light yet filling lunch ideas that are perfect for weight loss:

1. Grilled Chicken and Quinoa Bowl
   - Ingredients: Grilled chicken breast, cooked quinoa, mixed greens, cherry tomatoes, cucumber, avocado, lemon vinaigrette.
   - Instructions: In a bowl, layer the mixed greens, quinoa, and grilled chicken slices. Top with cherry tomatoes, cucumber slices, and avocado. Drizzle with lemon vinaigrette and serve.

2. Turkey and Avocado Wrap

- Ingredients: Whole-grain tortilla, sliced turkey breast, avocado, spinach, tomato, mustard or hummus.
- Instructions: Spread mustard or hummus on the tortilla. Layer with turkey slices, avocado, spinach, and tomato. Roll up the tortilla and slice in half.

3. Veggie and Hummus Plate
- Ingredients: Assorted raw vegetables (carrots, bell peppers, cucumber, cherry tomatoes), hummus, whole-grain crackers.
- Instructions: Arrange the vegetables on a plate with a serving of hummus in the center. Add a few whole-grain crackers on the side for a balanced meal.

4. Salmon and Asparagus Salad
- Ingredients: Grilled salmon, asparagus, mixed greens, cherry tomatoes, red onion, balsamic vinaigrette.
- Instructions: Place the mixed greens on a plate. Top with grilled salmon, steamed

asparagus, cherry tomatoes, and red onion slices. Drizzle with balsamic vinaigrette.

5. Stuffed Bell Peppers
   - Ingredients: Bell peppers, lean ground turkey or beef, quinoa, black beans, corn, diced tomatoes, shredded cheese.
   - Instructions: Preheat the oven to 375°F (190°C). Cut the tops off the bell peppers and remove the seeds. In a skillet, cook the ground turkey or beef. Mix in the quinoa, black beans, corn, and diced tomatoes. Stuff the mixture into the bell peppers, top with shredded cheese, and bake for 20-25 minutes.

Salads and Soups for Weight Loss

Salads and soups are excellent choices for a weight-loss-friendly lunch. They can be packed with nutrients, low in calories, and very satisfying.

Salads

1. Greek Salad

   - Ingredients: Cucumber, cherry tomatoes, red onion, Kalamata olives, feta cheese, bell pepper, mixed greens, olive oil, lemon juice, oregano.

   - Instructions: Chop the vegetables and mix them with mixed greens. Add olives and feta cheese. Drizzle with olive oil and lemon juice, then sprinkle with oregano.

2. Kale and Quinoa Salad

   - Ingredients: Kale, cooked quinoa, dried cranberries, toasted almonds, goat cheese, olive oil, lemon juice, honey.

   - Instructions: Massage the kale with a little olive oil to soften. Mix in the quinoa, dried cranberries, and toasted almonds. Top with crumbled goat cheese. For the dressing, whisk together olive oil, lemon juice, and honey.

3. Asian Chicken Salad

   - Ingredients: Grilled chicken breast, shredded cabbage, carrots, bell peppers, edamame, green onions, sesame seeds, Asian dressing (soy sauce, sesame oil, rice vinegar, honey).

- Instructions: Toss the shredded cabbage, carrots, bell peppers, and edamame together. Top with grilled chicken slices, green onions, and sesame seeds. Drizzle with Asian dressing.

Soups

1. Lentil Soup
   - Ingredients: Lentils, carrots, celery, onion, garlic, diced tomatoes, vegetable broth, spinach, cumin, paprika.
   - Instructions: In a large pot, sauté onion, garlic, carrots, and celery. Add lentils, diced tomatoes, and vegetable broth. Bring to a boil, then simmer until lentils are tender. Add spinach and season with cumin and paprika.

2. Chicken and Vegetable Soup
   - Ingredients: Chicken breast, carrots, celery, onion, garlic, zucchini, green beans, chicken broth, thyme, bay leaves.
   - Instructions: In a pot, cook chicken breast in broth until done, then shred. Sauté onion, garlic, carrots, and celery in a separate pan. Add

shredded chicken, zucchini, green beans, and broth. Season with thyme and bay leaves, then simmer until vegetables are tender.

3. Tomato Basil Soup
   - Ingredients: Tomatoes, onion, garlic, fresh basil, vegetable broth, olive oil, salt, pepper.
   - Instructions: Sauté onion and garlic in olive oil. Add tomatoes and broth, then simmer. Blend the soup until smooth, then stir in fresh basil. Season with salt and pepper.

Protein-Packed Lunches

For a lunch that keeps you full and satisfied, incorporate high-quality proteins. Here are some protein-packed lunch recipes:

1. Tuna Salad with Avocado
   - Ingredients: Canned tuna, avocado, Greek yogurt, celery, red onion, lemon juice, salt, pepper.
   - Instructions: In a bowl, mix drained tuna with diced avocado, Greek yogurt, chopped celery,

and red onion. Season with lemon juice, salt, and pepper. Serve on whole-grain bread or with a side of vegetables.

2. Chicken and Black Bean Bowl
   - Ingredients: Grilled chicken breast, black beans, brown rice, corn, salsa, avocado, cilantro.
   - Instructions: In a bowl, layer brown rice, black beans, corn, and grilled chicken. Top with salsa, diced avocado, and chopped cilantro.

3. Egg Salad Lettuce Wraps
   - Ingredients: Hard-boiled eggs, Greek yogurt, Dijon mustard, green onions, lettuce leaves, salt, pepper.
   - Instructions: Mash hard-boiled eggs with Greek yogurt and Dijon mustard. Add chopped green onions and season with salt and pepper. Serve in large lettuce leaves as wraps.

4. Tofu and Vegetable Stir-Fry
   - Ingredients: Firm tofu, broccoli, bell peppers, snap peas, carrots, soy sauce, ginger, garlic, sesame oil.

- Instructions: Press and cube the tofu, then stir-fry in sesame oil until golden. Add chopped vegetables and stir-fry until tender. Add soy sauce, grated ginger, and minced garlic. Serve over brown rice or quinoa.

5. Turkey Meatballs with Zoodles
  - Ingredients: Ground turkey, egg, breadcrumbs, garlic, parsley, zucchini, marinara sauce, Parmesan cheese.
  - Instructions: Mix ground turkey with egg, breadcrumbs, garlic, and parsley. Form into meatballs and bake at 400°F (200°C) until cooked through. Spiralize zucchini into zoodles and lightly sauté. Serve meatballs over zoodles with marinara sauce and a sprinkle of Parmesan cheese.

These lunch recipes are designed to provide a balance of nutrients, keeping you full and energized throughout the day. They focus on lean proteins, whole grains, and plenty of vegetables, supporting your weight loss journey while offering delicious and satisfying meals.

CHAPTER 6:

DINNER RECIPES

Satisfying Dinner Recipes

Dinner is an important meal that should be both satisfying and nutritious. Here are some wholesome dinner ideas that are filling and flavorful:

1. Grilled Lemon Herb Chicken with Roasted Vegetables
  - Ingredients: Chicken breast, lemon juice, olive oil, garlic, rosemary, thyme, assorted vegetables (carrots, bell peppers, zucchini, broccoli), salt, pepper.
  - Instructions: Marinate chicken in lemon juice, olive oil, garlic, rosemary, and thyme for at least 30 minutes. Grill the chicken until fully cooked. Toss vegetables in olive oil, salt, and pepper, and roast at 400°F (200°C) for 20-25

minutes. Serve the chicken with the roasted vegetables.

2. Baked Salmon with Asparagus and Quinoa
   - Ingredients: Salmon filets, asparagus, quinoa, olive oil, garlic, lemon, dill, salt, pepper.
   - Instructions: Preheat the oven to 375°F (190°C). Place salmon and asparagus on a baking sheet, drizzle with olive oil, and season with garlic, lemon juice, dill, salt, and pepper. Bake for 15-20 minutes. Cook quinoa according to package instructions. Serve salmon and asparagus over quinoa.

3. Stuffed Bell Peppers
   - Ingredients: Bell peppers, lean ground beef or turkey, quinoa, black beans, corn, tomato sauce, shredded cheese.
   - Instructions: Preheat the oven to 375°F (190°C). Cut the tops off the bell peppers and remove the seeds. In a skillet, cook the ground meat and mix in cooked quinoa, black beans, corn, and tomato sauce. Stuff the mixture into

the bell peppers, top with shredded cheese, and bake for 25-30 minutes.

4. Shrimp Stir-Fry
  - Ingredients: Shrimp, mixed vegetables (broccoli, bell peppers, snap peas, carrots), soy sauce, garlic, ginger, sesame oil.
  - Instructions: In a wok or large pan, heat sesame oil and sauté garlic and ginger. Add shrimp and cook until pink. Add vegetables and stir-fry until tender-crisp. Add soy sauce and stir well. Serve over brown rice or noodles.

5. Chicken and Vegetable Skewers
  - Ingredients: Chicken breast, bell peppers, onions, zucchini, cherry tomatoes, olive oil, garlic, Italian seasoning, salt, pepper.
  - Instructions: Preheat the grill. Cut chicken and vegetables into chunks. In a bowl, mix olive oil, garlic, Italian seasoning, salt, and pepper. Thread chicken and vegetables onto skewers, brush with the marinade, and grill until chicken is cooked through.

Low-Carb and High-Protein Dinners

Low-carb and high-protein dinners can help with weight loss and muscle maintenance. Here are some delicious options:

1. Cauliflower Rice Stir-Fry with Beef
   - Ingredients: Ground beef, cauliflower rice, bell peppers, onions, garlic, soy sauce, ginger, sesame oil.
   - Instructions: In a large pan, cook ground beef until browned. Add onions, garlic, and bell peppers, and sauté until tender. Stir in cauliflower rice, soy sauce, and ginger. Cook until cauliflower rice is tender. Drizzle with sesame oil before serving.

2. Zucchini Noodles with Pesto and Grilled Chicken
   - Ingredients: Zucchini (spiralized into noodles), chicken breast, pesto sauce, cherry tomatoes, pine nuts, Parmesan cheese.
   - Instructions: Grill the chicken breast and slice. In a pan, lightly sauté zucchini noodles

with a little olive oil until tender. Toss with pesto sauce and cherry tomatoes. Top with grilled chicken slices, pine nuts, and Parmesan cheese.

3. Baked Cod with Lemon and Herbs
   - Ingredients: Cod filets, lemon, garlic, parsley, olive oil, salt, pepper.
   - Instructions: Preheat the oven to 400°F (200°C). Place cod filets in a baking dish, drizzle with olive oil, and season with minced garlic, chopped parsley, salt, and pepper. Top with lemon slices and bake for 15-20 minutes. Serve with a side of steamed vegetables.

4. Turkey and Spinach Stuffed Portobello Mushrooms
   - Ingredients: Ground turkey, spinach, Portobello mushrooms, garlic, onion, marinara sauce, mozzarella cheese, Italian seasoning.
   - Instructions: Preheat the oven to 375°F (190°C). Remove stems from mushrooms and set aside. In a pan, cook ground turkey with garlic, onion, and spinach. Add marinara sauce and Italian seasoning. Stuff the mushrooms with

the mixture, top with mozzarella cheese, and bake for 15-20 minutes.

5. Eggplant Lasagna
  - Ingredients: Eggplant, ground turkey or beef, marinara sauce, ricotta cheese, mozzarella cheese, Parmesan cheese, Italian seasoning.
  - Instructions: Preheat the oven to 375°F (190°C). Slice eggplant into thin rounds and bake for 10 minutes. In a pan, cook ground meat with marinara sauce and Italian seasoning. In a baking dish, layer eggplant slices, meat sauce, ricotta cheese, and mozzarella cheese. Repeat layers and top with Parmesan cheese. Bake for 25-30 minutes.

Vegetarian and Vegan Options

For those following a vegetarian or vegan diet, these dinner recipes are nutrient-dense and satisfying:

1. Chickpea and Vegetable Curry

- Ingredients: Chickpeas, coconut milk, diced tomatoes, mixed vegetables (carrots, bell peppers, spinach), curry powder, garlic, ginger, onion, rice.
- Instructions: In a pot, sauté onion, garlic, and ginger. Add curry powder and cook briefly. Add diced tomatoes, coconut milk, chickpeas, and mixed vegetables. Simmer until vegetables are tender. Serve over rice.

2. Stuffed Sweet Potatoes
- Ingredients: Sweet potatoes, black beans, corn, avocado, cherry tomatoes, cilantro, lime juice, salt, pepper.
- Instructions: Preheat the oven to 400°F (200°C). Bake sweet potatoes until tender. In a bowl, mix black beans, corn, diced avocado, cherry tomatoes, chopped cilantro, lime juice, salt, and pepper. Cut the sweet potatoes in half and top with the mixture.

3. Quinoa and Black Bean Stuffed Bell Peppers

- Ingredients: Bell peppers, quinoa, black beans, corn, diced tomatoes, onion, garlic, cumin, chili powder, avocado.
- Instructions: Preheat the oven to 375°F (190°C). Cut the tops off the bell peppers and remove the seeds. In a pan, sauté onion and garlic, then add quinoa, black beans, corn, diced tomatoes, cumin, and chili powder. Stuff the mixture into the bell peppers and bake for 25-30 minutes. Top with diced avocado.

4. Vegan Lentil Shepherd's Pie
- Ingredients: Lentils, mixed vegetables (carrots, peas, corn), onion, garlic, vegetable broth, mashed potatoes (made with almond milk and olive oil), salt, pepper.
- Instructions: Preheat the oven to 375°F (190°C). In a pan, sauté onion and garlic, then add lentils, mixed vegetables, and vegetable broth. Cook until vegetables are tender. Spread the mixture in a baking dish and top with mashed potatoes. Bake for 20-25 minutes until the top is golden.

5. Vegetable Stir-Fry with Tofu

   - Ingredients: Firm tofu, broccoli, bell peppers, snap peas, carrots, soy sauce, garlic, ginger, sesame oil, brown rice or noodles.

   - Instructions: Press and cube the tofu, then stir-fry in sesame oil until golden. Add chopped vegetables and stir-fry until tender. Add soy sauce, grated ginger, and minced garlic. Serve over brown rice or noodles.

These dinner recipes offer a variety of flavors and nutrients to support a balanced diet. Whether you're looking for low-carb, high-protein, vegetarian, or vegan options, these meals are designed to be satisfying and conducive to weight loss and overall health.

CHAPTER 7:

SNACKS AND APPETIZERS

Healthy Snack Options

Snacking can be a healthy part of your diet if you choose nutrient-dense options. Here are some snacks that are not only healthy but also help keep you full and satisfied:

1. Greek Yogurt with Berries and Nuts
   - Ingredients: Greek yogurt, mixed berries (blueberries, strawberries, raspberries), almonds or walnuts, honey (optional).
   - Instructions: Combine Greek yogurt with a handful of mixed berries and nuts. Drizzle with honey if desired.

2. Hummus and Vegetable Sticks
   - Ingredients: Hummus, carrots, cucumber, bell peppers, celery.

- Instructions: Slice vegetables into sticks and serve with a portion of hummus for dipping.

3. Apple Slices with Almond Butter
   - Ingredients: Apple, almond butter, cinnamon (optional).
   - Instructions: Slice the apple and spread almond butter on each slice. Sprinkle with cinnamon if desired.

4. Mixed Nuts and Seeds
   - Ingredients: Almonds, walnuts, sunflower seeds, pumpkin seeds.
   - Instructions: Mix a handful of nuts and seeds for a crunchy, protein-rich snack.

5. Rice Cakes with Avocado and Cherry Tomatoes
   - Ingredients: Rice cakes, avocado, cherry tomatoes, salt, pepper.
   - Instructions: Mash avocado and spread it on rice cakes. Top with halved cherry tomatoes, and season with salt and pepper.

Fat-Burning Appetizers

These appetizers contain ingredients known for their fat-burning properties, making them a great addition to a weight-loss-friendly diet:

1. Spicy Edamame
   - Ingredients: Edamame (in pods), olive oil, garlic, chili flakes, salt.
   - Instructions: Boil edamame until tender. In a pan, heat olive oil and sauté minced garlic and chili flakes. Toss in the edamame and stir until coated. Season with salt and serve warm.

2. Cucumber and Smoked Salmon Bites
   - Ingredients: Cucumber, smoked salmon, cream cheese, dill, lemon zest.
   - Instructions: Slice cucumber into rounds. Top each slice with a small dollop of cream cheese, a piece of smoked salmon, and a sprinkle of dill and lemon zest.

3. Stuffed Mushrooms

- Ingredients: Button mushrooms, garlic, spinach, feta cheese, olive oil, breadcrumbs (optional).

- Instructions: Preheat oven to 375°F (190°C). Remove stems from mushrooms and set aside. Sauté minced garlic and spinach in olive oil. Mix with crumbled feta cheese and breadcrumbs if using. Stuff the mixture into mushroom caps and bake for 15-20 minutes.

4. Guacamole with Veggie Chips

- Ingredients: Avocado, lime juice, red onion, cilantro, jalapeño, salt, assorted vegetable chips.

- Instructions: Mash avocado and mix with lime juice, finely chopped red onion, cilantro, diced jalapeño, and salt. Serve with vegetable chips.

5. Buffalo Cauliflower Bites

- Ingredients: Cauliflower florets, hot sauce, olive oil, garlic powder, paprika, salt.

- Instructions: Preheat oven to 400°F (200°C). Toss cauliflower florets in a mixture of hot sauce, olive oil, garlic powder, paprika, and salt.

Spread on a baking sheet and bake for 20-25 minutes, until crispy.

Quick and Easy Snacks

These snacks are perfect for when you're short on time but still want something healthy and delicious:

1. Banana and Peanut Butter
   - Ingredients: Banana, natural peanut butter.
   - Instructions: Slice the banana and spread peanut butter on each slice.

2. Trail Mix
   - Ingredients: Dried fruits (raisins, cranberries, apricots), mixed nuts, dark chocolate chips.
   - Instructions: Combine a handful of dried fruits, nuts, and dark chocolate chips for a quick energy boost.

3. Protein Balls
   - Ingredients: Rolled oats, peanut butter, honey, protein powder, chia seeds.

- Instructions: Mix all ingredients until well combined. Roll into small balls and refrigerate until firm.

4. Veggie Roll-Ups
  - Ingredients: Whole-grain tortilla, hummus, sliced cucumber, bell peppers, spinach.
  - Instructions: Spread hummus on the tortilla, layer with sliced vegetables, and roll up. Slice into bite-sized pieces.

5. Hard-Boiled Eggs
  - Ingredients: Eggs, salt, pepper.
  - Instructions: Boil eggs for 9-12 minutes, then peel. Slice in half and season with salt and pepper.

These snacks and appetizers are designed to be both nutritious and satisfying, helping you manage your hunger between meals and supporting your weight loss goals. They focus on whole foods, healthy fats, and proteins to keep you energized and full.

CHAPTER 8:

DESSERTS AND SWEETS

Guilt-Free Dessert Recipes

Enjoying dessert doesn't have to mean straying from your healthy eating goals. Here are some guilt-free dessert recipes that satisfy your sweet tooth while keeping nutrition in mind:

1. Chia Seed Pudding
   - Ingredients: Chia seeds, almond milk (or any milk of choice), vanilla extract, honey or maple syrup, fresh berries.
   - Instructions: Mix chia seeds with almond milk, vanilla extract, and a sweetener. Refrigerate for at least 4 hours or overnight until it thickens. Top with fresh berries before serving.

2. Baked Apples with Cinnamon
   - Ingredients: Apples, cinnamon, honey or maple syrup, chopped nuts (optional).

- Instructions: Preheat the oven to 350°F (175°C). Core the apples and place them in a baking dish. Sprinkle with cinnamon and drizzle with honey. Bake for 20-25 minutes until tender. Top with chopped nuts if desired.

3. Greek Yogurt and Fruit Parfait
   - Ingredients: Greek yogurt, mixed fresh fruit (berries, kiwi, mango), granola (optional), honey.
   - Instructions: Layer Greek yogurt with fresh fruit and granola in a glass. Drizzle with honey and serve immediately.

4. Frozen Banana Bites
   - Ingredients: Bananas, dark chocolate (70% cocoa or higher), crushed nuts or coconut flakes.
   - Instructions: Slice bananas and dip in melted dark chocolate. Place on a baking sheet lined with parchment paper and sprinkle with crushed nuts or coconut flakes. Freeze until the chocolate is set.

5. Avocado Chocolate Mousse

- Ingredients: Ripe avocados, cocoa powder, honey or maple syrup, vanilla extract.
- Instructions: Blend ripe avocados with cocoa powder, honey, and vanilla extract until smooth. Chill before serving.

Healthy Alternatives to Traditional Sweets

Replacing traditional sweets with healthier alternatives can help you enjoy the flavors you love without compromising on nutrition. Here are some delicious alternatives:

1. Almond Flour Brownies
   - Ingredients: Almond flour, cocoa powder, eggs, coconut oil, honey or maple syrup, vanilla extract.
   - Instructions: Preheat the oven to 350°F (175°C). Mix almond flour, cocoa powder, eggs, melted coconut oil, sweetener, and vanilla extract. Pour into a baking pan and bake for 20-25 minutes.

2. Fruit Sorbet

- Ingredients: Frozen fruit (such as mango, berries, or peaches), a splash of lemon or lime juice, a touch of honey (optional).
- Instructions: Blend frozen fruit with lemon or lime juice and a bit of honey if needed. Serve immediately or freeze until firm.

3. Oatmeal Cookies
- Ingredients: Rolled oats, mashed banana, almond butter, raisins or dark chocolate chips, cinnamon.
- Instructions: Preheat the oven to 350°F (175°C). Mix oats, mashed banana, almond butter, raisins or chocolate chips, and cinnamon. Drop spoonfuls of the mixture onto a baking sheet and bake for 10-12 minutes.

4. Pumpkin Spice Energy Balls
- Ingredients: Pumpkin puree, oats, almond butter, pumpkin pie spice, honey.
- Instructions: Mix all ingredients together, roll into small balls, and refrigerate until firm.

5. Apple Nachos

- Ingredients: Apple slices, almond butter, dark chocolate chips, chopped nuts, a sprinkle of cinnamon.
- Instructions: Arrange apple slices on a plate. Drizzle with almond butter and sprinkle with dark chocolate chips, chopped nuts, and a bit of cinnamon.

Low-Sugar Dessert Options

For those looking to reduce sugar intake, these low-sugar dessert options are perfect:

1. Berry Compote
  - Ingredients: Mixed berries (fresh or frozen), a splash of lemon juice, a small amount of honey or stevia (optional).
  - Instructions: Cook berries with lemon juice over medium heat until they break down into a sauce. Sweeten with a small amount of honey or stevia if desired.

2. Coconut Milk Ice Cream

- Ingredients: Coconut milk, vanilla extract, a small amount of honey or stevia, a pinch of salt.
  - Instructions: Mix coconut milk with vanilla extract, sweetener, and salt. Pour into an ice cream maker and churn according to the manufacturer's instructions.

3. Baked Pears with Walnuts
  - Ingredients: Pears, chopped walnuts, cinnamon, a drizzle of honey (optional).
  - Instructions: Preheat the oven to 350°F (175°C). Halve and core the pears. Place in a baking dish, sprinkle with cinnamon and walnuts, and bake for 20-25 minutes. Drizzle with honey if desired.

4. Raspberry Chia Jam
  - Ingredients: Fresh or frozen raspberries, chia seeds, a small amount of honey or stevia.
  - Instructions: Cook raspberries until they break down. Stir in chia seeds and sweetener, and cook for an additional 5 minutes. Let cool before using.

5. Cinnamon Baked Almonds

   - Ingredients: Raw almonds, cinnamon, a touch of honey or stevia.

   - Instructions: Preheat the oven to 350°F (175°C). Toss almonds with cinnamon and a small amount of honey or stevia. Spread on a baking sheet and bake for 10-12 minutes, stirring occasionally.

These dessert options allow you to indulge your sweet tooth while maintaining a focus on health and nutrition. They provide alternatives that are lower in sugar and higher in beneficial nutrients, helping you stay on track with your weight loss goals.

CHAPTER 9:

DRINKS AND SMOOTHIES

Hydration and Its Role in Weight Loss

Proper hydration is crucial for overall health and effective weight management. Here's how staying hydrated can support your weight loss journey:

1. Metabolism Boost: Drinking enough water can increase your metabolic rate, helping your body burn calories more efficiently.

2. Appetite Control: Sometimes, thirst is mistaken for hunger. Staying hydrated helps prevent unnecessary snacking.

3. Detoxification: Water helps flush out toxins from your body, which can improve your overall health and support weight loss.

4. Digestive Health: Adequate hydration supports proper digestion and helps prevent constipation.

5. Exercise Performance: Staying hydrated improves physical performance, making it easier to stay active and burn calories.

Fat-Burning Drinks

Incorporating fat-burning drinks into your daily routine can enhance your weight loss efforts. Here are some drinks known for their metabolism-boosting and fat-burning properties:

1. Green Tea
   - Ingredients: Green tea leaves or tea bags, hot water, lemon (optional).
   - Instructions: Steep green tea leaves or a tea bag in hot water for 3-5 minutes. Add a squeeze of lemon for extra flavor and benefits.

2. Apple Cider Vinegar Drink

- Ingredients: Apple cider vinegar, water, lemon juice, honey (optional).
- Instructions: Mix 1-2 tablespoons of apple cider vinegar with a glass of water. Add a splash of lemon juice and honey if desired. Drink before meals.

3. Cucumber Mint Water
- Ingredients: Cucumber, fresh mint leaves, water.
- Instructions: Slice cucumber and add to a pitcher of water with mint leaves. Let infuse in the refrigerator for a few hours before drinking.

4. Ginger Lemon Detox Drink
- Ingredients: Fresh ginger, lemon, hot water, honey (optional).
- Instructions: Slice fresh ginger and steep in hot water. Add lemon juice and honey if desired. Drink warm or chilled.

5. Matcha Tea
- Ingredients: Matcha powder, hot water, almond milk (optional).

- Instructions: Whisk matcha powder into hot water until frothy. Add almond milk if desired for a creamy texture.

Smoothie Recipes for Weight Loss

Smoothies can be a convenient and delicious way to support weight loss. Here are some healthy smoothie recipes designed to keep you satisfied and boost your metabolism:

1. Green Detox Smoothie
   - Ingredients: Spinach, kale, green apple, cucumber, lemon juice, ginger, water.
   - Instructions: Blend a handful of spinach and kale with a chopped green apple, cucumber, lemon juice, and a small piece of ginger. Add water to achieve desired consistency.

2. Berry Protein Smoothie
   - Ingredients: Mixed berries (blueberries, strawberries, raspberries), Greek yogurt, protein powder, almond milk.

- Instructions: Blend a cup of mixed berries with a scoop of protein powder, a dollop of Greek yogurt, and almond milk. Adjust the consistency with more almond milk if needed.

3. Avocado and Banana Smoothie
   - Ingredients: Ripe avocado, banana, spinach, almond milk, chia seeds.
   - Instructions: Blend half an avocado with a banana, a handful of spinach, almond milk, and a tablespoon of chia seeds.

4. Tropical Weight Loss Smoothie
   - Ingredients: Pineapple, mango, coconut water, lime juice, a handful of spinach.
   - Instructions: Blend pineapple, mango, and spinach with coconut water and a splash of lime juice.

5. Chocolate Almond Smoothie
   - Ingredients: Almond butter, unsweetened cocoa powder, banana, almond milk, a pinch of cinnamon.

- Instructions: Blend almond butter with cocoa powder, a banana, almond milk, and a pinch of cinnamon.

These drink and smoothie recipes are designed to be nutrient-dense, hydrating, and supportive of your weight loss goals. They offer a variety of flavors and health benefits, helping you stay on track while enjoying delicious beverages.

CHAPTER 10:

SPECIAL DIET CONSIDERATIONS

Gluten-Free Options

For those with gluten intolerance or celiac disease, these gluten-free recipes and tips can help you stay on track while avoiding gluten:

1. Quinoa Salad with Vegetables
   - Ingredients: Quinoa, cherry tomatoes, cucumber, bell peppers, red onion, feta cheese (optional), lemon vinaigrette.
   - Instructions: Cook quinoa according to package instructions and let it cool. Combine with chopped vegetables and feta cheese. Dress with lemon vinaigrette.

2. Sweet Potato and Black Bean Tacos

- Ingredients: Sweet potatoes, black beans, corn tortillas, avocado, salsa, cilantro.
- Instructions: Roast sweet potatoes until tender. Warm corn tortillas and fill with sweet potatoes, black beans, avocado slices, salsa, and cilantro.

3. Chia Seed Pudding

- Ingredients: Chia seeds, almond milk, vanilla extract, fresh fruit.
- Instructions: Mix chia seeds with almond milk and vanilla extract. Refrigerate overnight until it thickens. Top with fresh fruit before serving.

4. Baked Salmon with Asparagus

- Ingredients: Salmon filets, asparagus, olive oil, garlic, lemon juice, salt, pepper.
- Instructions: Preheat oven to 375°F (190°C). Place salmon and asparagus on a baking sheet, drizzle with olive oil and lemon juice, and season with garlic, salt, and pepper. Bake for 15-20 minutes.

5. Almond Flour Pancakes
   - Ingredients: Almond flour, eggs, baking powder, almond milk, vanilla extract.
   - Instructions: Mix almond flour with eggs, baking powder, almond milk, and vanilla extract. Cook on a griddle until golden brown on both sides.

Dairy-Free Recipes

For those avoiding dairy, these recipes are both delicious and free from dairy products:

1. Coconut Milk Smoothie
   - Ingredients: Coconut milk, frozen berries, banana, spinach.
   - Instructions: Blend coconut milk with frozen berries, banana, and a handful of spinach until smooth.

2. Avocado and Tomato Salad
   - Ingredients: Avocado, cherry tomatoes, red onion, cilantro, lime juice, olive oil.

- Instructions: Dice avocado and tomatoes. Combine with chopped red onion and cilantro. Dress with lime juice and olive oil.

3. Cauliflower Rice Stir-Fry
  - Ingredients: Cauliflower rice, mixed vegetables, soy sauce, garlic, ginger, sesame oil.
  - Instructions: Sauté garlic and ginger in sesame oil, add vegetables and cauliflower rice, and stir-fry until tender. Season with soy sauce.

4. Sweet Potato and Kale Soup
  - Ingredients: Sweet potatoes, kale, vegetable broth, onions, garlic, cumin.
  - Instructions: Sauté onions and garlic, add diced sweet potatoes and vegetable broth, and cook until potatoes are tender. Stir in kale and cumin before serving.

5. Chickpea and Spinach Curry
  - Ingredients: Chickpeas, spinach, coconut milk, curry powder, onions, garlic.
  - Instructions: Sauté onions and garlic, add chickpeas, curry powder, and coconut milk.

Simmer until heated through and stir in spinach before serving.

Low-Carb and Keto-Friendly Foods

For those following a low-carb or ketogenic diet, these recipes focus on high-fat, low-carb ingredients:

1. Zucchini Noodles with Pesto
   - Ingredients: Zucchini (spiralized), pesto sauce, cherry tomatoes, Parmesan cheese (optional).
   - Instructions: Sauté zucchini noodles until tender. Toss with pesto sauce and cherry tomatoes. Top with Parmesan cheese if desired.

2. Stuffed Bell Peppers
   - Ingredients: Bell peppers, ground beef or turkey, cauliflower rice, diced tomatoes, cheese (optional).
   - Instructions: Preheat oven to 375°F (190°C). Cook ground meat with cauliflower rice and diced tomatoes. Stuff the mixture into halved

bell peppers and bake until peppers are tender. Top with cheese if desired.

3. Egg Salad Lettuce Wraps
   - Ingredients: Eggs, mayonnaise, Dijon mustard, lettuce leaves, chives.
   - Instructions: Chop hard-boiled eggs and mix with mayonnaise, Dijon mustard, and chives. Serve wrapped in lettuce leaves.

4. Keto Chicken Salad
   - Ingredients: Cooked chicken, avocado, celery, mayonnaise, lemon juice, salt, pepper.
   - Instructions: Combine chopped chicken with diced avocado, celery, mayonnaise, and lemon juice. Season with salt and pepper.

5. Bacon-Wrapped Asparagus
   - Ingredients: Asparagus spears, bacon, olive oil, garlic powder.
   - Instructions: Wrap asparagus spears with bacon slices and place on a baking sheet. Drizzle with olive oil and sprinkle with garlic powder. Bake at 400°F (200°C) for 15-20 minutes.

These recipes accommodate various dietary needs, ensuring you can enjoy delicious meals while adhering to gluten-free, dairy-free, and low-carb or keto diets. Each option is designed to be both flavorful and aligned with specific dietary restrictions.

CHAPTER 11:

LIFESTYLE TIPS FOR SUSTAINABLE WEIGHT LOSS

Mindful Eating Practices

Mindful eating involves paying full attention to the experience of eating and drinking, both inside and outside the body. This practice can enhance your relationship with food and help with weight management:

1. Eat Slowly and Without Distractions
   - Focus on your food by eating slowly and avoiding distractions like television or smartphones. This helps you savor your meals and recognize your body's hunger and fullness cues.

2. Listen to Your Body

- Pay attention to hunger and satiety signals. Eat when you're truly hungry and stop when you're comfortably full, rather than when your plate is empty or because it's time to eat.

3. Enjoy Each Bite
   - Take the time to appreciate the flavors, textures, and aromas of your food. Chew thoroughly and savor each bite, which can help you feel more satisfied with smaller portions.

4. Practice Portion Control
   - Serve smaller portions to avoid overeating. Use smaller plates and bowls to help manage portion sizes and reduce the temptation to go back for seconds.

5. Keep a Food Journal
   - Record what you eat and drink, including your emotions and hunger levels. This can help you identify patterns, make more mindful choices, and stay accountable.

Importance of Sleep and Stress Management

Adequate sleep and effective stress management are crucial for maintaining a healthy weight and overall well-being:

1. Prioritize Quality Sleep
  - Aim for 7-9 hours of quality sleep per night. Poor sleep can disrupt hormones that regulate hunger and appetite, leading to increased cravings and weight gain.

2. Develop a Consistent Sleep Routine
  - Go to bed and wake up at the same time every day, even on weekends. Create a relaxing pre-sleep routine to signal your body that it's time to wind down.

3. Manage Stress Effectively
  - Chronic stress can lead to emotional eating and weight gain. Practice stress-relief techniques such as meditation, deep breathing exercises, or yoga to help manage stress levels.

4. Engage in Regular Physical Activity

 - Regular exercise not only supports weight loss but also helps improve sleep quality and reduce stress. Find activities you enjoy and make them a regular part of your routine.

5. Seek Support When Needed
 - If stress or sleep issues are impacting your health, consider talking to a healthcare provider or therapist for guidance and support.

Building Healthy Habits

Developing sustainable habits is key to long-term weight management and overall health. Here are strategies for building and maintaining healthy habits:

1. Set Realistic Goals
 - Set achievable and specific goals for yourself. Break them into smaller, manageable steps to make progress feel more attainable and less overwhelming.

2. Create a Routine

- Establish a daily routine that incorporates healthy habits, such as meal planning, regular exercise, and adequate hydration. Consistency is key to making these habits stick.

3. Stay Hydrated
   - Drink plenty of water throughout the day to support metabolism, digestion, and overall health. Carry a water bottle with you as a reminder to stay hydrated.

4. Plan and Prepare Meals
   - Plan your meals and snacks in advance to avoid reaching for unhealthy options. Prepare healthy meals and snacks ahead of time to make nutritious choices easier.

5. Find Support and Accountability
   - Share your goals with friends, family, or a support group to stay motivated. Having someone to share your journey with can provide encouragement and accountability.

6. Celebrate Progress

- Recognize and celebrate your achievements, no matter how small. Rewarding yourself for reaching milestones can help maintain motivation and reinforce positive behavior.

By incorporating mindful eating practices, prioritizing sleep and stress management, and building healthy habits, you can create a sustainable approach to weight loss and overall wellness. These lifestyle changes will support not just short-term goals but long-term health and well-being.

CHAPTER 12:

TRACKING YOUR PROGRESS

Keeping a Food Journal

Maintaining a food journal can be a powerful tool for tracking your dietary habits and supporting weight loss. Here's how to effectively keep a food journal:

1. Record Everything You Eat and Drink
   - Write down all meals, snacks, and beverages, including portion sizes and preparation methods. This helps you become more aware of your eating patterns.

2. Note Your Emotions and Hunger Levels
   - Document your mood and hunger levels before and after eating. This can help identify emotional eating triggers and patterns.

3. Use Technology
  - Consider using food tracking apps or digital journals for convenience and ease. Many apps can also analyze nutritional information and track your progress.

4. Review and Reflect
  - Regularly review your food journal to identify trends and areas for improvement. Reflect on what's working well and what needs adjustment.

5. Stay Honest and Consistent
  - Be honest and consistent with your entries. Accurate tracking will provide a clearer picture of your dietary habits and progress.

Setting Realistic Goals

Setting achievable and realistic goals is essential for long-term success in weight management. Here's how to set effective goals:

1. Make Goals Specific and Measurable
   - Define clear, specific goals that are measurable. For example, "Lose 5 pounds in 1 month" or "Eat vegetables with every meal."

2. Set Short-Term and Long-Term Goals
   - Create both short-term (weekly or monthly) and long-term (quarterly or yearly) goals. Short-term goals help maintain motivation, while long-term goals provide a broader perspective.

3. Ensure Goals Are Attainable
   - Set goals that are realistic and achievable based on your current lifestyle and resources. Avoid setting goals that are too ambitious or unrealistic.

4. Create a Plan of Action
   - Develop a detailed plan for how you will achieve each goal. Break down the steps required and establish a timeline for reaching them.

5. Monitor and Adjust Goals
   - Regularly assess your progress toward your goals and adjust them as needed. If you encounter obstacles, modify your plan to stay on track.

Adjusting Your Diet for Continued Success

Adapting your diet over time can help ensure ongoing progress and prevent plateaus. Here's how to adjust your diet effectively:

1. Evaluate Your Progress Regularly
   - Review your food journal and assess your progress toward your goals. Identify any patterns or areas where you may need to make changes.

2. Modify Your Caloric Intake
   - If weight loss stalls, consider adjusting your caloric intake. Reduce or increase your calories slightly to match your current weight loss needs.

3. Incorporate New Foods and Recipes

- Introduce new, healthy foods and recipes to keep your diet interesting and nutritionally balanced. Experiment with different fruits, vegetables, and lean proteins.

4. Adjust Macronutrient Ratios
   - If needed, adjust the balance of macronutrients (carbohydrates, proteins, and fats) in your diet based on your progress and how your body is responding.

5. Seek Professional Advice
   - Consult a registered dietitian or nutritionist for personalized advice and adjustments. They can provide expert guidance tailored to your individual needs.

By effectively tracking your progress, setting realistic goals, and making necessary adjustments to your diet, you can maintain momentum and achieve sustained success in your weight loss journey. These practices will help you stay focused, motivated, and on track toward your long-term health and wellness goals.

CHAPTER 13:

SUCCESS STORIES AND TESTIMONIALS

Real-Life Examples of Weight Loss Without Exercise

Inspiration can often be found in the stories of those who have achieved weight loss through dietary changes alone. Here are a few real-life examples:

1. John's Journey to Better Health
   - Background: John, a 45-year-old office worker, struggled with weight due to a sedentary lifestyle and poor eating habits.
   - Approach: He focused on reducing processed foods and increasing his intake of whole foods, such as lean proteins, vegetables, and healthy fats.

- Results: John lost 30 pounds over six months by making dietary changes, including portion control and mindful eating. His blood sugar levels improved, and he felt more energetic.

2. Maria's Transformation
   - Background: Maria, a 32-year-old mother of two, needed to lose weight to improve her overall health and energy levels.
   - Approach: She adopted a low-carb, high-protein diet, emphasizing foods like eggs, leafy greens, and lean meats. She also incorporated more hydration and mindful eating practices.
   - Results: Maria lost 20 pounds in four months, experienced reduced cravings, and found greater satisfaction with her meals. Her confidence and energy levels increased significantly.

3. Tom's Weight Loss Success
   - Background: Tom, a 50-year-old who had been struggling with his weight for years, decided to make changes after experiencing health issues.

- Approach: Tom focused on a balanced diet, emphasizing whole grains, lean proteins, and plenty of vegetables. He also tracked his food intake and made adjustments based on his progress.

- Results: Tom lost 40 pounds over eight months, improved his cholesterol levels, and felt more active and healthier overall.

Tips and Advice from Success Stories

Here are some valuable tips and advice derived from successful weight loss journeys without exercise:

1. Prioritize Whole Foods
- Focus on incorporating nutrient-dense, whole foods into your diet. Avoid processed and high-sugar foods that can lead to weight gain and poor health.

2. Practice Portion Control
- Be mindful of portion sizes to avoid overeating. Use smaller plates, measure

servings, and listen to your body's hunger and fullness cues.

3. Stay Consistent

- Consistency is key to long-term success. Stick to your dietary plan and make gradual adjustments as needed. Consistent habits yield better results over time.

4. Track Your Progress

- Keep a food journal or use a tracking app to monitor your dietary habits and progress. This helps identify patterns, make informed adjustments, and stay accountable.

5. Incorporate Mindful Eating

- Focus on eating slowly and enjoying your meals. Mindful eating can help you feel more satisfied with smaller portions and reduce emotional eating.

6. Stay Hydrated

- Drink plenty of water throughout the day to support metabolism, digestion, and overall health. Hydration can also help control hunger and prevent overeating.

7. Seek Support
   - Share your goals with friends, family, or a support group. Having a support system can provide encouragement, accountability, and motivation.

Motivation and Encouragement

Maintaining motivation throughout your weight loss journey is crucial for success. Here's some encouragement to keep you on track:

1. Celebrate Small Wins
   - Recognize and celebrate each milestone, no matter how small. Achieving small goals can boost your confidence and keep you motivated.

2. Focus on Health, Not Just Weight
   - Shift your focus from just losing weight to improving overall health and well-being. Pay attention to how dietary changes are positively

impacting your energy levels, mood, and health markers.

3. Remember Your "Why"
   - Keep in mind the reasons you started your weight loss journey, whether it's for better health, increased energy, or improved self-confidence. Revisiting your motivations can help you stay focused.

4. Stay Positive
   - Maintain a positive mindset and be kind to yourself. Understand that setbacks are a normal part of the process. Learn from them and keep moving forward.

5. Inspire Others
   - Share your success and experiences with others who may be on a similar journey. Your story can inspire and encourage others to make positive changes in their lives.

By learning from real-life success stories, incorporating practical tips, and staying motivated, you can achieve your weight loss goals and maintain a healthier lifestyle without the need for exercise.

CONCLUSION

Recap of Key Points

In this book, we've explored effective strategies for losing weight without exercise, focusing on the pivotal role of diet in weight management. Here's a summary of the key points:

1. The Science of Weight Loss:
   - Understanding how the body burns fat, the importance of a balanced diet, and debunking common myths about weight loss.

2. Foods That Burn Fat:
   - Incorporating thermogenic foods and a variety of fat-burning foods such as lean proteins, whole grains, fruits, vegetables, and healthy fats into your diet.

3. Meal Planning and Preparation:

- The significance of meal planning, tips for effective meal prep, and sample meal plans tailored for weight loss.

4. Breakfast, Lunch, and Dinner Recipes:
   - Quick and nutritious breakfast options, light and filling lunch ideas, satisfying dinner recipes, and low-carb and high-protein meals.

5. Snacks, Appetizers, Desserts, and Drinks:
   - Healthy snack options, fat-burning appetizers, guilt-free desserts, and smoothies designed for weight loss.

6. Special Diet Considerations:
   - Gluten-free, dairy-free, and low-carb or keto-friendly food options to accommodate various dietary needs.

7. Lifestyle Tips for Sustainable Weight Loss:
   - Mindful eating practices, the importance of sleep and stress management, and strategies for building healthy habits.

8. Tracking Your Progress:
   - Keeping a food journal, setting realistic goals, and adjusting your diet for continued success.

9. Success Stories and Testimonials:
   - Real-life examples of weight loss without exercise, tips and advice from successful individuals, and motivational encouragement.

Final Tips for Long-Term Success

To ensure lasting success in your weight loss journey, consider these final tips:

1. Maintain Consistency:
   - Consistency is key to achieving and maintaining weight loss. Stick to your dietary plan and make healthy choices a part of your daily routine.

2. Adapt and Evolve:
   - Be open to making adjustments as needed. Evolving your diet and habits in response to

your progress and changing needs can help you stay on track.

3. Prioritize Self-Care:
- Take care of your physical and mental health. Prioritizing self-care can enhance your overall well-being and support your weight management goals.

4. Stay Educated:
- Keep learning about nutrition and healthy eating. Staying informed can help you make better choices and adapt to new information.

5. Celebrate Achievements:
- Regularly recognize and celebrate your progress. Celebrating your successes, both big and small, can boost motivation and reinforce positive behavior.

Encouragement to Begin Your Journey

Embarking on a weight loss journey without exercise is a commendable step toward improving your health and well-being. Remember that success is built on small, consistent changes and a positive mindset. Start by implementing the strategies outlined in this book and tailor them to fit your personal needs and preferences.

Your journey is unique, and every step forward is a step toward achieving your goals. Stay motivated, be patient with yourself, and embrace the process. With dedication and the right approach, you can achieve lasting weight loss and enjoy a healthier, more fulfilling life.

Now is the perfect time to begin your journey. Take the first step today and embrace the changes that will lead you to success. Your future self will thank you for the commitment and effort you invest now.

www.ingramcontent.com/pod-product-compliance
Lightning Source LLC
Chambersburg PA
CBHW050808250726
48653CB00006B/2140